Yoga Beyond the Poses

Esoteric YOGA

*The Ultimate Beginner's Guide
to Discover the Secrets of Yoga,
Sex Magic, and Magical Mantras!*

Shreyanada Natha

Illustrator
Mattias Långström

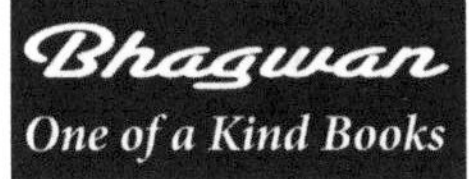

Esoteric

YOGA

*The Ultimate Beginner's Guide
to Discover the Secrets of Yoga,
Sex Magic, and Magical Mantras!*

Shreyanada Natha

ISBN 9789198839272

✳✳✳

Copyright © Mattias Långström

2 FREE PREMIUM BONUS!

#1. Download the **AUDIOBOOK** *at the back of the book!*

#2. Download **CHAKRA-INDEX IN COLOR** *here!*

SCAN QR-CODE or go to:

https://bit.ly/47wdFVZ

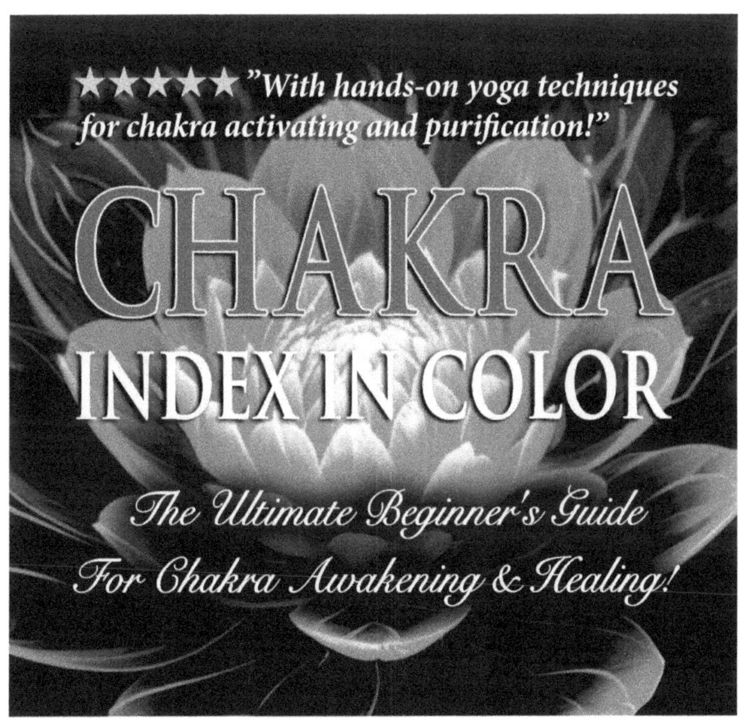

FREE PREMIUM Audiobook
Authentic Yoga Nidra Meditation
Sahasrara Chakra Awakening!

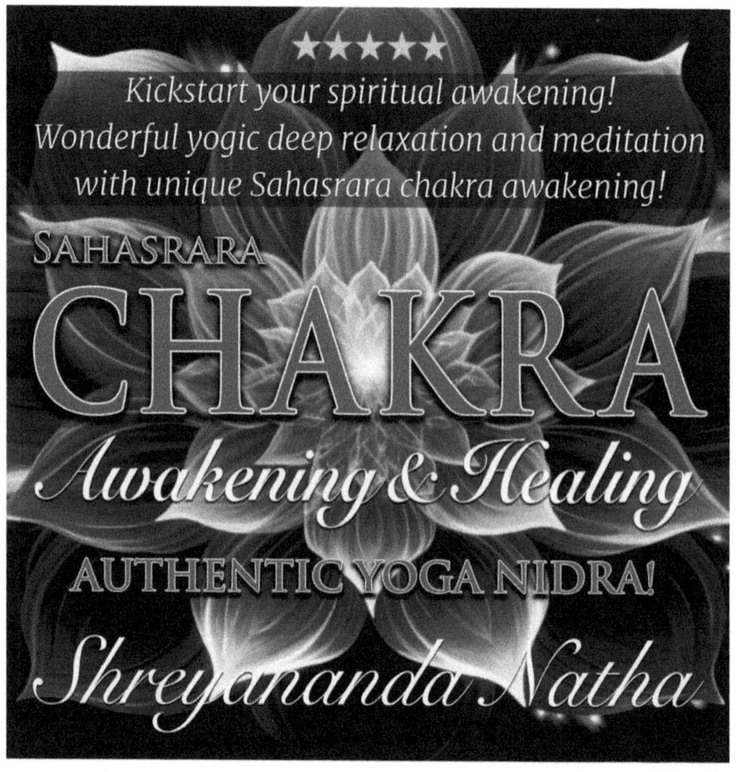

Download the **AUDIOBOOK** at the back of the book!

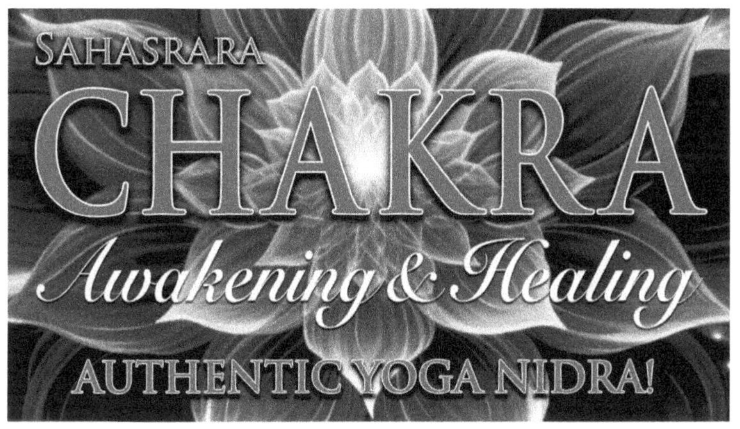

Kickstart your spiritual awakening! Wonderful yogic deep relaxation and meditation with unique Sahasrara chakra awakening and healing.

PRESENTATION

Yoga Nidra, or yogic sleep, is a unique meditation process that's powerfully profound and healing for body, mind, and spirit.

Practitioners are led into a state of deep relaxation and the experience of our chakra system.

Yoga Nidra offers extensive benefits, yet it is one of the most straightforward yoga practices.

All you have to do is put on your most comfortable clothes, find a quiet space, lie down on your back, and play the meditation.

Yoga Beyond the Poses – Esoteric Yoga
The Ultimate Beginner's Guide to Discover the Secrets of Yoga, Sex Magic, and Magical Mantras!
Including A Premium Audiobook: Yoga Nidra Meditation – Sahasrara Chakra Awakening And Healing!

The book describes Esoteric yoga and the secrets of yoga. Read about sex magic, secret chakras, and magical mantras! It penetrates deeply but remains easy to read, educational, and understandable. A must on the bookshelf for anyone interested in Esoteric yoga and who quickly wants to know more. The ultimate magic book for beginners!

The book is part of a series of seven yoga books, Yoga Beyond the Poses: The Ultimate Beginner's Guide to Yoga, that delve into the seven key areas of yoga.

INCLUDING A PREMIUM AUDIOBOOK: AUTHENTIC YOGA NIDRA MEDITATION – SAHASRARA CHAKRA AWAKENING & HEALING!
Kickstart your spiritual awakening! Wonderful yogic deep relaxation and meditation with unique Sahasrara chakra awakening and healing.

Yoga Nidra, or yogic sleep, is a unique meditation process that's powerfully profound and healing for body, mind, and spirit. Practitioners are led into a state of deep relaxation

and the experience of our chakra system. Yoga Nidra offers extensive benefits, yet it is one of the most straightforward yoga practices. All you have to do is put on your most comfortable clothes, find a quiet space, lie down on your back, and play the meditation. –
Download the audiobook at the back of the book!

ABOUT THE BOOK SERIES
YOGA BEYOND THE POSES: *The Ultimate Beginner's Guide to Yoga!*

The book is part of a seven-book yoga series, Yoga Beyond the Poses: The Ultimate Beginner's Guide to Yoga, that delve into yoga's seven most important areas. They are straightforward to read, educational, and fascinating. A must on the bookshelf for anyone interested in yoga who quickly wants to know more.

MY NAME AND MY MISSION
Shreyananda Natha was the name I was given when I was initiated into the Natha Order and received the master mantra – the Shodasi mantra, after studying yoga and tantra for over twelve years, the highest mantra in yoga and tantra. It means "he who knows".

After practicing yoga and meditation continuously for over twenty years, having a yoga school for many years, and leading studies for yoga teachers, I wanted to get out more wi-

dely with yoga into our whole society, out of the small yoga room. Spread the knowledge of yoga, our chakra system, and Kundalini Shakti to anyone who will listen. What needed to be added were educational fact books on yoga that didn't just skim the surface or deal with the author's private life. So it became my Sankalpa, my magical wish, and my mission to create exciting yoga books that everyone should be able to read and enjoy. To show how we can apply and use yoga in different areas of life and achieve success and health. Here and now.

If you like my books, feel free to follow me on my social media, share and like, tell your friends about the books, and write an honest review; one or two lines don't matter. All support is precious.

Thanks!

THE AUTHOR

Shreyananda Natha is the author of popular and best-selling yoga books. He has, among other things, written one of the most comprehensive books about yoga – EVERYTHING ABOUT YOGA and the study book – TEACHING YOGA AND MEDITATION BEYOND THE POSES. He is also a certified yoga and meditation teacher according to the EYTF international guidelines. He has undergone multi-year yoga teacher training under the guidance of Swami Omananda at Satyananda Ashram and holds the highest initiation in the tantric Natha order. He frequently travels to Asia and India to learn and gain knowledge and inspiration. He has immersed himself in tantric rituals and is known for his extensive knowledge of yoga, deep relaxation, and meditation.

"There is no authority that can say what yoga is. When you surrender yourself completely and fully and experience yoga without limitations and doubts, the true encounter with yoga occurs when you become one with the true experience within you. Only then will you understand what yoga is – for you. When you are no longer limited by neatness, shyness, and artificial thought patterns that act as a filter between you and the transformation. Yoga is a cultural-historical wealth still passed on from teacher to student and helps man find his way back to his true nature. It opens us up and attracts awareness. It strengthens our self-esteem, and our person's entire spectrum of possibilities suddenly becomes visible.

Yoga is not difficult or strange. You don't have to become a vegan, a monk, or be able to stand on your head. You just need to do your yoga regularly; the rest will take care of itself. You can use yoga and meditation to feel better, both physically and mentally, but also to achieve success and develop in all areas of life – here and now."

Good luck!

Namasté

I want to thank the teachers and students I've had over the years who have made my journey with yoga so enjoyable. Thank you for all the inspiration you have given me and for making this book possible. The yoga masters who no longer live among us – live on with each new person who immerses themselves in the yoga tradition.

Sri Swami Sivananda, Sri Swami Satyananda, Sri Tirumalai Krishnamacharya, Sri Swami Vishnudevananda, Sri K. Pattabhi Jois, Osho, Swami Nirdosha, Swami Omananda, Swami Janakananda, Ole Schmidt, Turiya, Maryam Abrishami and Sanna Kuittinen.

People who all searched for answers to what they sensed through an activated Ajna chakra. In yoga, they have learned the principles behind the universe, the collective consciousness, and the creative force, Kundalini Shakti. The duality behind everything, both what we see and what we don't see. Together, we are helped to pass on the previously secret knowledge about our gunas, nadis, and chakras to all who want to become a Rishi.

Aum Shri Durgayai Namaha

Shreyananda Natha

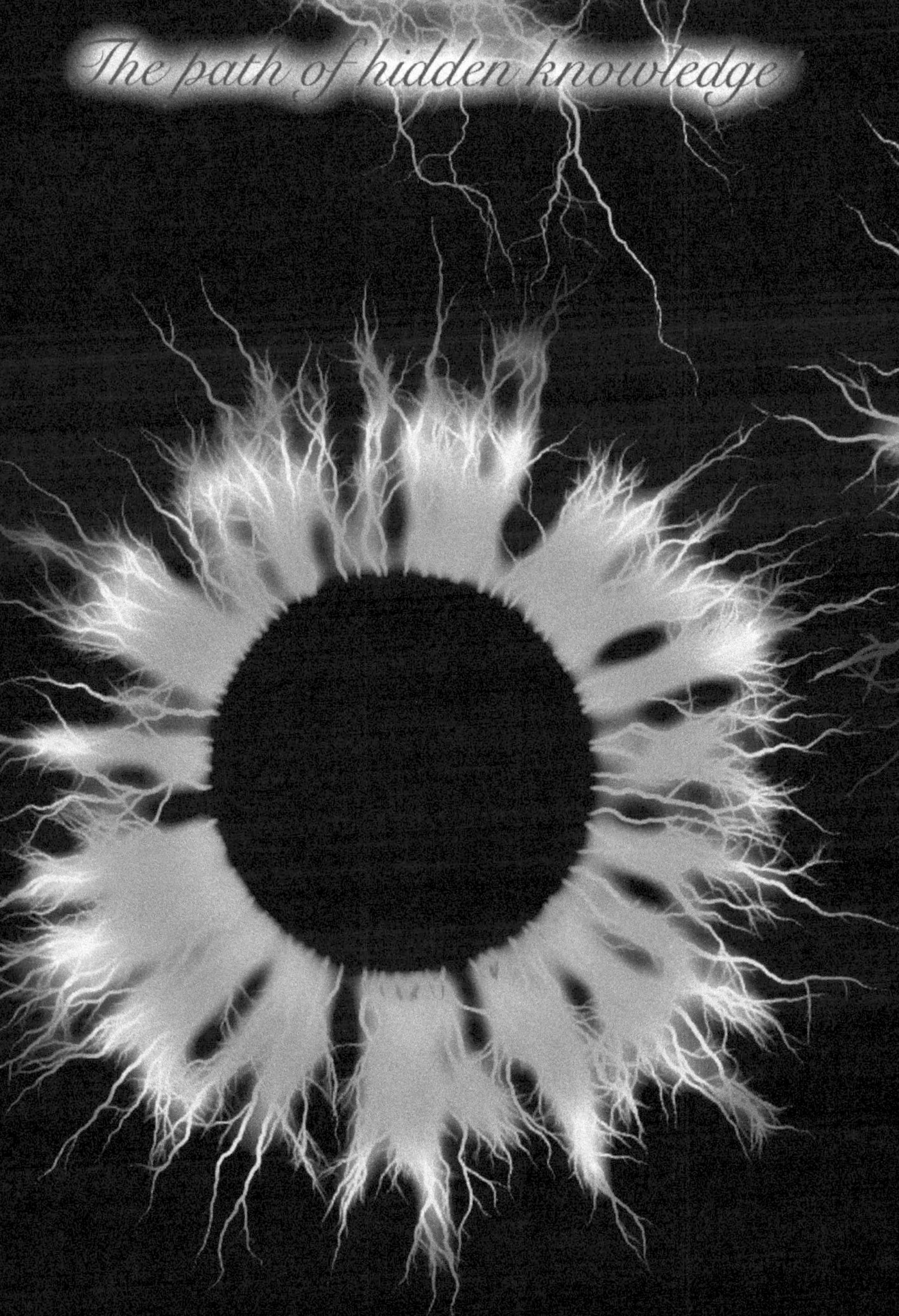

ESOTERIC YOGA
The path of hidden knowledge
ESOTERIC YOGA
The path of hidden knowledge

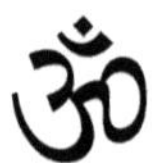

ESOTERIC YOGA

THE WAY OF HIDDEN KNOWLEDGE

Esoteric means "inaccessible" or "only for the initiated" and is most often used to denote the hidden wisdom or secret spiritual knowledge that underlies philosophical systems. The term esoteric can also refer to the teachings and practices of supersensible experiences that require special preparation and training, often under the guidance of an experienced teacher.

One might wonder why knowledge is hidden. The answer is multifaceted, but in addition to the fact that the mysterious and hidden have an appeal to new students, it has a purely practical explanation. For example, if someone is only temporarily curious, they will most likely forget a mantra told to them, even if it could be life-saving. Tradition – the knowledge of it – will go nowhere. On the other hand, if a person undergoes demanding yogic and tantric training for years, that person will be more likely to remember the mantra. Keeping the knowledge hidden ensures that it is passed on and preserved for the future.

According to an old prophecy, the hidden, esoteric, tantric acts would one day be practiced quite openly – during Kali's age – which is now. It allows me to write about the most advanced tantric rituals previously hidden. However, I can not reveal everything. I can not tell you everything about things that can be abused. For example, I will not show the most potent mantra there is, the Shodasi mantra. A mantra that can replace all other secret mantras and gives the holder the power to influence everything in the macro and microcosm: the power of life and death, success and defeat. However, I can tell you about other previously hidden ones, the rituals that are refined through training and give the adept an increased awareness and vitality to successfully deal with everything in life. There is no point in not telling about that knowledge, in not passing it on. It would be like not telling interested people where they can find the best running shoes. Everything that can make it easier for people to have increased vitality and joy in life must now be acknowledged. The time has come. The time is now. The time is yours. Good luck!

THE PATH OF THE RIGHT AND LEFT HANDS

In tantra, the basis of all yoga, the hidden knowledge is preserved in two directions or paths: the path of the right hand (dakshinachara) and the path of the left hand (vamachara). Both paths aim to awaken Kundalini Shakti and give the practitioner cosmic power. Both paths are considered equal ways of enlightening the Indian tantric practitioners, although vamachara is regarded as the faster and more dangerous way.

DAKSHINACHARA

Dakshinachara is also described as the inner way or the path of meditation. Rituals are based on the practitioner's inner meditation, such as Kriya yoga.

VAMACHARA

Vamachara, the path of external meditation, is often the path that people know in tantra, where the adept gets help from things and experiences in the outside world to expand power—for example, the use of meat and wine in the maithuna ritual (tantric intercourse).

Both paths use secret mantras and yantras in their tantric rituals to achieve their purposes.

MANTRA SHASTRA

Mantra shastra is the foundation of all spiritual practice and is central to all esoteric yoga.

MANTRA

The most basic mantra is Aum, also known as the pranava mantra, the source of all mantras.

Two types of mantras which have a literal meaning are:

1.) SAGUNA MANTRA

Mantras that represent and invoke a deity, God, or goddess for spiritual self-realization. Saguna mantras create visual patterns through repeated chanting until the deity appears appropriately.

Some examples of saguna mantras are:

a) Om Namah Shivaya. Greetings to Shiva.
b) Om Nam Narayanaya. Greetings to God over harmony and balance.
c) Gayatri mantra. Dedicated to the goddess Gayatri.
d) Mahamrityunjaya mantra. Dedicated to Shiva.

More similar mantras are shanti mantra, Ram, Sita, Om Aing Saraswati Namaha, etc.

2.) NIRGUNA MANTRA

Mantras that are formless, abstract, and represent the universe as a whole and not in any specific form are called nirguna mantras. These mantras require a higher form of concentration as they do not refer to any actual form. They are for more profound meditation, and with regular practice, siddhis (paranormal abilities) are obtained.

The use of nirguna mantras is primarily to become one with the absolute or to identify with the divine in the universe.

Some examples of nirguna mantras are:

a) Om (Aum).
Om is the original mantra, the root of all sounds and letters that create language and thoughts.
b) So Ham.

We unconsciously utter this mantra every time we breathe. On inhalation – So, and on exhalation – Ham. So Ham means – I am that, beyond the limitations of the mind and body, I am one with the infinite. I am. That's me.

There are primarily ten different types of magic mantras without a literal meaning:

1. Shanti (Siddhi) mantra – to free oneself from disease, fear, imagination, and other problems.

2. Stambhan's mantra is to make living beings unable to move.

3. Mohana mantra – used to create attraction.

4. The Uchchatan mantra is used to create mental imbalances in people.

5. Vashikaran mantra – used to turn someone into an enslaved person.

6. The Akarshan mantra is used to acquire wealth and material happiness.

7. The Jrambhan mantra is used to change human behavior.

8. The Vidweshan mantra is used to make two people enemies.

9. Maran mantra – used to kill someone.

10. The Paustik mantra is used to become successful on all levels.

SRI YANTRA

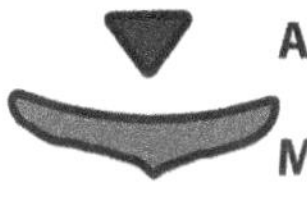
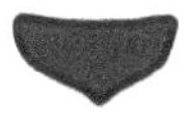
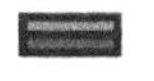

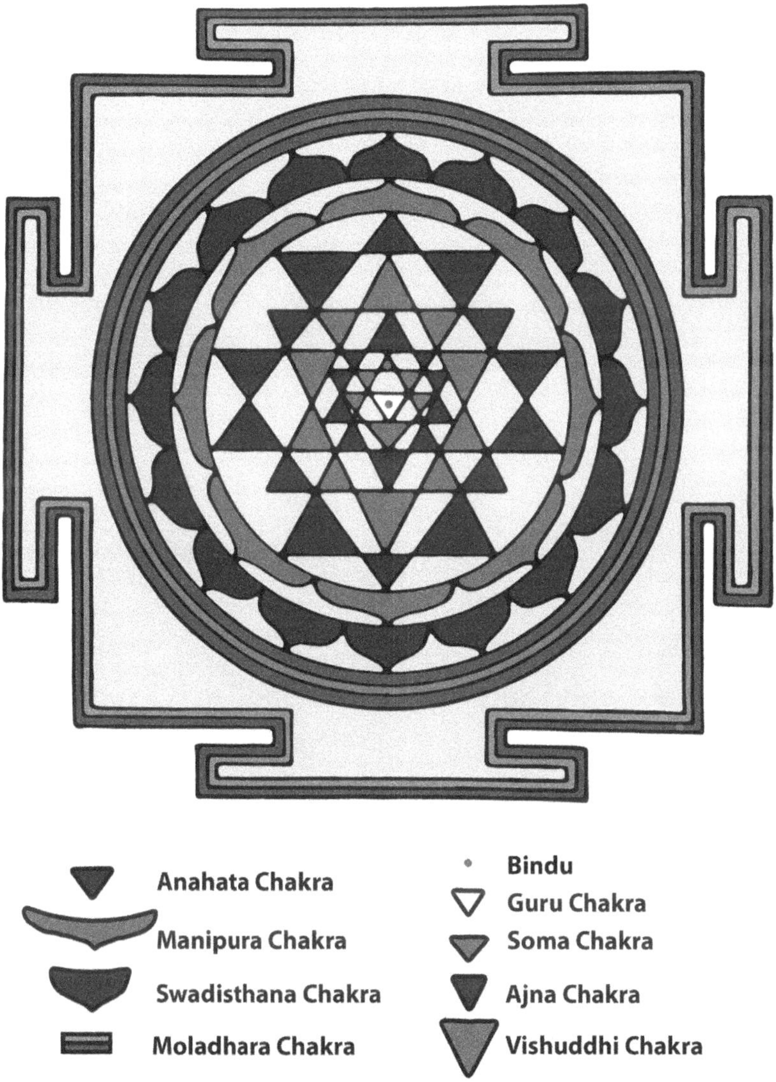

Anahata Chakra

Manipura Chakra

Swadisthana Chakra

Moladhara Chakra

Bindu

Guru Chakra

Soma Chakra

Ajna Chakra

Vishuddhi Chakra

SRI VIDYA MANTRA – SHODASI MANTRA

Sri Yantra – also known as Sri Chakra – is the mother of all yantras because all others are descended from it. It is the most potent yantra and symbolizes the creation of the cosmos and all life. Sri Vidya is worshiped by the tantric of both the right and left hands.

Sri Vidya or Sri Chakra represents Sri Lalita or Tripura Sundari – Shakti in her most beautiful form, a sixteen-year-old beauty. Sixteen syllables represent Sri Lalita as she is also associated with sixteen desires.

Since Sri Yantra is the most potent yantra, it also possesses the most powerful mantra – the Shodasi mantra. It is logical if you think about it, as each form also has a sound.

The Shodasi mantra is the most secret and protected and is impossible to find out about – unless a guru initiates you. Forget all the internet pages claiming to know the mantra because it is entirely wrong and unreasonable. If you have undergone all the trials that it means to be initiated, you do not give it away – especially not on the internet.

Typically, one does not initiate the Shodasi mantra directly; the guru decides which time and place is most favorable. Generally, you are first started in the Bala mantra, then depending on your maturity and insight, you are initiated in the Panchadasi mantra. The Panchadasi mantra is a mantra made up of fifteen stages syllables. If the guru thinks the adept is ready for final liberation, he is initiated into the shodasi mantra and gains knowledge of the secret sixteenth stage.

For the adept to achieve complete liberation and obtain magical abilities, so-called siddhis, he must recite the mantra nine hundred thousand times and add purascharana each time at the end.

BRAHMA VIDYA – THE BIGGEST SECRET

Shodashi vidya is also called Brahma vidya: Brahman (the world soul) and Vidya (the knowledge). Brahman is rendered into mantra form in Shodasi vidya, and because of this, it is guarded as the greatest secret.

Suppose the practitioner can reach the fourth level of consciousness, turiya (superconsciousness). In that case, he is most likely prepared to go beyond this to get the fifth level of consciousness, turiyatita. Turiyatita can be achieved without difficulty when the Shodasi mantra is recited regularly.

Therefore, you become one with Brahman by reaching turiyatita (the fifth level of consciousness) and reciting the shodasi mantra. There is nothing after this.

What happens when a person is transformed into turiyatita? The world soul, the divine consciousness, replaces the soul. You become divine and gain divine power.

24

It is also something that can be experienced in a moment of near death; a person is never the same after such an experience.

BIJA MANTRA

Mantras often used in tantra are bija mantras. They are different sounds that have no direct literal meaning, but that has the power to create a significant transformation and expansion of the physical, emotional, and mental forces. They are called bija mantras, or so-called magical sounds.

The approximately fifty sacred sounds from the Sanskrit alphabet (bija mantras) are primarily resonants for the seven major chakras. Correctly stated, they activate the energy in different chakras and purify and balance the mind and body. They also increase the power of various mantra compositions.

AIM

After Om (Aum), the second most common bija mantra is Aim, pronounced – Aym. The Aim is the feminine aspect of Om and often follows Om in various mantras. Om and Aim consist of two compound vowels, including all sounds.

Om helps to purify the mind, and Aim helps to focus in different ways.

Just as Om is the sound of the invisible, Aim is the sound of the visible. Om is the sound of the unmanifested, and Aim is the sound of the manifested. The principle of consciousness and energy. Shiva and Shakti. Therefore, one can often hear

Aim in Shakti mantras. Mantras of the Divine Mother. The Aim is the bija mantra for Saraswati, the goddess of knowledge and speech. Aim helps us in education, art, expression, and communication and is suitable for all forms of school work in general. The Aim is also a guru mantra and helps us to have more excellent knowledge of everything. It also helps us with concentration during the recitation of the mantras.

HRIM

After Om and Aim, Hrim pronounced "Hreem," the most common bija mantra. It combines the sound Ha, which stands for energy / prana, space, and light, with the sound of Ra, which stands for fire, light, and learning, and the sound A, which stands for energy, concentration, and motivation.

Hrim is bija mantra for Shakti or Parvati.

Hrim is a mantra for magic, attraction, love, and power. It brings us joy, ecstasy, passion, and complete happiness.

Hrim is a specific mantra for the heart (hridaya in Sanskrit) on all its levels: spiritually, emotionally, as a chakra, and as a physical organ.

SRIM

Srim, pronounced "Shreem," is one of the most common bija mantras due to its favorable properties. It attracts everything that is good and favorable and helps us develop positively. Srim is the bija mantra of Lakshmi and is also called the Ramas bija when used to worship Lord Rama.

Srim is the mantra of faith, devotion, refuge, and surrender. It can be used to take shelter in or indulge in various deities and obtain their favors.

Srim relates to the heart more from a feminine and senti-mental perspective, while Hrim relates to the heart from a masculine, pranic, or functional perspective.

Srim is often used with Hrim as Hrim relates to the sun, and Srim relates to the moon.

KRIM

Krim is pronounced "Kreem," the most crucial bija mantra that begins with a harsh consonant. Krim begins with Ka, the first consonant in Sanskrit, which shows manifested pra-na and the initial energy phase. To Ka, it adds the Ra sound of fire and the A sound that concentrates power like the other Shakti mantras. Krim creates light just like Hrim and Srim but on a more specific and actualized level.

Krim is the bija mantra of Kali, the goddess of time, destruc-tion, and transformation. Kali also creates the highest energy level within us.

Krim is the mantra of work, yoga, and the energy of trans-formation. It is known to be a bija mantra for yoga practitioners and is applied to awaken Kundalini Shakti within us. Krim stimulates higher perceptiveness and prana and stabilizes pratyahara within us. The mantra can create contact with any deity.

KLIM

Klim is pronounced "Kleem" and is the softer, more feminine aspect of Krim. Just as Krim is electric, Klim is magnetic and attracts things to us.

Klim relates to Akarshana Shakti or the law of attraction. Klim is the bija mantra for Krishna and Sundari, the goddesses of love and beauty. It is also the bija mantra over all desires (kama bija) and helps us achieve our inner desires. Klim is the mantra of love and devotion and increases the level of love within us. Because of this, it is one of the most used mantras.

STRIM

Strim, pronounced "Streem," is composed of the Sa sound, which stands for stability, and the Ta sound, which creates expansion, with the A sound, which provides us with energy, direction, and motivation.

Strim is known to be the peace mantra, the so-called shanti bija. The mantra Strim provides the power to have children, enrich something nutritionally, protect, and guide. It is similar to Srim but more robust and has a more stabilizing effect.

Strim is the bija mantra of the Hindu goddess Tara (not the Buddhist Tara). Hindu Tara is associated with Durga, often called Durga-Tara, a guarding and protective form of the goddess.

HUM

Hum is pronounced "Hoom" and is one of the most essential bija mantras, along with Om, Aim, and Hrim. It is said to be Pranava, the sound of Lord Shiva.

Hum is the great agni or fire mantra and can increase the fire within us at all levels—everything from the fire of consciousness to the pranic fire to the burning of the body.

Hum is also a weapon, a protecting mantra that can destroy negativity with its enlightening fire. It is also called the bija mantra of anger (krodha bija).

Hum relates to a violent form of the goddess, like Kali, Chandi or Chinnamasta.

Hum raises Kundalini Shakti with breathing and concentration on the navel (Manipura chakra).

THE SECRET CHAKRAS

In yoga, people usually talk about seven or eight more signi-ficant chakras along the spine and at the top of the head. If you count Bindu visarga as a chakra, you say that a human has eight major vital chakras. According to popular belief, Bindu is located on the top of the back of the head and has no kshetram.

In the hidden tradition, you learn a big secret: Bindu's place-ment on the back of the head is the chakra's kshetram. That Bindu is located above the Sahasrara chakra and is called Sunya. When the Kundalini Shakti reaches the Sunya – the black chakra, one is transformed into a deity and receives divine qualities.

In addition to Sunya, other chakras are hidden: Guru, Nir-vana, Indu, Manas, and Tala (Lalana) chakras are placed in the head, and Hrit chakra is placed just below the Anahata chakra, the heart chakra.

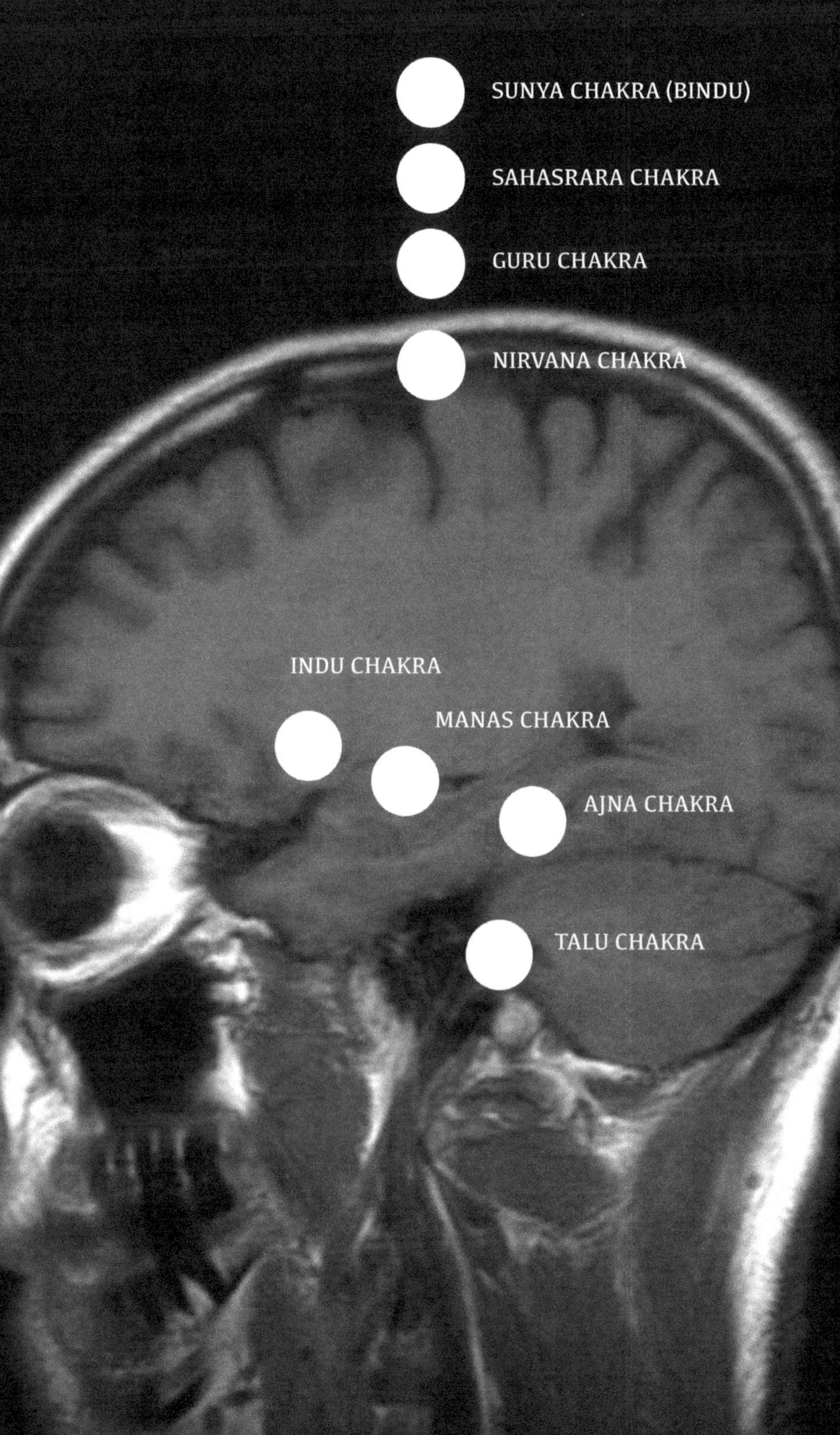

SUNYA CHAKRA (BINDU)
SAHASRARA CHAKRA
GURU CHAKRA
NIRVANA CHAKRA
INDU CHAKRA
MANAS CHAKRA
AJNA CHAKRA
TALU CHAKRA

THE HIDDEN RITUALS

KRIYA YOGA

There are seventy-two kriyas, of which twenty are the most used and suitable for daily use by any student. These kriyas are divided into three groups:

1. Those who evoke pratyahara.
2. Those who evoke dharana.
3. Those that induce dhyana.

KRIYAS FOR PRATYAHARA:

VIPAREETA KARANI MUDRA

Come into vipareeta karani asana. Ensure the legs are straight and the chin does not touch the chest. Close your eyes and breathe ujjayi pranayama. Experience in an inhalation how the amrit or nectar flows along the spine from the Manipura to the Vishuddhi chakra and gathers there. Hold your breath for a while and experience how the nectar gets cool. Then, exhale with ujjayi breathing and experience how the nectar flows from Vishuddhi through Ajna, Bindu, and Sahasrara. After exhaling, take the consciousness to Manipura again and repeat the kriya twenty-one times.

CHAKRA ANUSANDHANA

Sit in a meditation position and close your eyes. Breathe

normally. Take consciousness to the Mooladhara chakra and follow the front passage "arohan" up to the Bindu. Repeat all the chakras up, Mooladhara, Swadhisthana, Manipura, Anahata, and Vishuddhi, and go from here directly to Bindu. Then, let the consciousness go down along the back passage and repeat the chakras on the way down. You are starting from Ajna, Vishuddhi, Anahata, Manipura, Swadhisthana, and Mooladhara. Then, start immediately on the next round, beginning with Swadhisthana. Please do not overdo it by trying to locate the chakras, but flow past them quickly. Practice nine rounds.

NADA SANCHALANA

Sit in a meditation position. Exhale completely. Open your eyes and bend your head down without pressing your chin against your chest. Take consciousness to the Mooladhara chakra. Silently repeat, "Mooladhara, Mooladhara, Mooladhara." Inhale and let the consciousness flow through the anterior passage "arohan" up to Bindu. Repeat the names of the chakras on the way up. When passing from Vishuddhi to Bindu, tilt your head slightly backward. Hold your breath and silently say "Bindu, Bindu, Bindu" to yourself. Then, continue down the back passage "awarohan" while saying the mantra Om inwardly. Close your eyes as you go down and experience the chakras. When you arrive at Mooladhara, hold your breath and repeat "Mooladhara" three times. Then, continue directly to the next round. Practice thirteen rounds.

PAWAN SANCHALANA

Sit in a meditation position and close your eyes. Practice khechari mudra and ujjayi pranayama. Exhale entirely and tilt your head down as in the previous kriya. Become aware of the Mooladhara chakra and silently repeat, "Mooladhara, Mooladhara, Mooladhara." Then inwardly say "arohan" and inhale with ujjayi breathing along the front passage while experiencing the chakras and mentally repeating their names. When you pass from Vishuddhi to Bindu, tilt your head back and silently repeat "Bindu, Bindu, Bindu." Then inwardly say "awarohan" and exhale along the back passage with ujjayi breathing. Repeat the name of the chakras silently and close your eyes slowly as you move down. Then open your eyes, tilt your head down, and start the next round. Practice forty-nine rounds.

SHABA SANCHALANA

Sit in a meditation position. Practice khechari mudra and ujjayi pranayama. Exhale entirely and open your eyes. Bend your head forward and pay attention to the Mooladhara chakra briefly. Inhale with ujjayi breathing and ascend along the anterior passage. Experience what the sound of breathing So sounds like on the way up. Experience each kshetram at the same time without any mental repetition. Tilt your head back at the transition from Vishuddhi to Bindu. Hold your breath and experience Bindu for a few seconds. Exhale, close your eyes, and hear the sound of the breath, Ham. Experience each chakra on the way down without rehearsing mentally. When you get to Mooladhara, open your eyes, bend your head, and start the next round. Practice fifty-nine rounds.

MAHA MUDRA

Sit in siddhasana or siddha yoni asana with your heel pressed against the Mooladhara. Practice khechari mudra, exhale entirely, and tilt your head forward. Keep your eyes open at first. Silently repeat, "Mooladhara, Mooladhara, Mooladhara." Climb upwards along the "arohan" with an ujjayi inhalation. Experience each kshetram on the way up. Raise your head as you pass from Vishuddhi to Bindu. At Bindu, repeat "Bindu, Bindu, Bindu" internally. Practice moola bandha and shambhavi mudra while holding your breath. Repeat mentally "shambhavi, kechari, mool". When you say "shambhavi", focus on the eyebrow center. When you say "kechari," focus on the tongue and palate. When you say "mool," focus on the Mooladhara chakra. Repeat this procedure thrice; accustomed practitioners repeat it twelve times—the first releases the shambhavi mudra and the moola bandha. Become aware of Bindu and walk down the back passage with ujjayi breathing to the Mooladhara chakra. Experience each chakra on the way down. With Mooladhara, tilt your head forward and open your eyes. Repeat "Mooladhara, Mooladhara, Mooladhara" and continue to the next round. Practice twelve rounds and finish with "Mooladhara, Mooladhara, Mooladhara".

MAHA BHEDA MUDRA

Sit as in the previous exercise. Practice khechari mudra and exhale completely. Keep your eyes open. Mentally repeat "Mooladhara, Mooladhara, Mooladhara." Inhale with ujjayi and ascend along the anterior passage to Bindu. As you pass from Vishuddhi to Bindu, lift your head. Repeat mentally, "Bindu, Bindu, Bindu." Go down the back passage to the Mooladhara with ujjayi breathing and close your eyes. Experience the chakras on the way down. Then, practice the jalandhara bandha while holding your breath. Practice nasikagra drishti, uddiyana bandha, and moola bandha. Mentally repeat "nasikagra, uddiyana, mool" and experience its seats in the body. Repeat the procedure three times as a beginner and twelve times when you are more accustomed. Release nasikagra drishti, moola bandha, uddiyana bandha and jalandhara bandha. Hold your head down and experience Mooladhara. Repeat "Mooladhara, Mooladhara, Mooladhara" mentally. Continue to the next round. Practice twelve rounds.

MANDUKI MUDRA

Sit in bhadrasana. Keep your eyes open. The body surface under the Mooladhara should be in contact with the floor. Place a pillow or blanket under you if necessary. Place your hands on your knees and practice nasikagra drishti. Become aware of the natural breath that flows through your nostrils. On inhalation, respiration flows through both nostrils and meets at the center of the eyebrows. On exhalation, the flow separates at the center of the eyebrows and through the nostrils—experience how breathing follows a V-shaped pattern. Be aware of all odors. The point of the kriya is to share the smell of the astral body, which is the smell of sandalwood. If your eyes get tired, close them for a while. Do the exercise until it feels intoxicating. Please do not get caught in it, but quit before you are absorbed by it too much.

TADAN KRIYA

Sit in padmasana with your eyes open. Place your hands next to your body on the floor with your fingers pointing forward. Tilt your head back and practice shambhavi mudra. Inhale through the mouth with ujjayi breathing. When you inhale, experience how the breathing sinks downwards through a tube between the mouth and the Mooladhara chakra. Hold your breath, experience the Mooladhara chakra, and practice the moola bandha. Using your hands, lift your body off the floor and lower it so the Mooladhara lightly hits the floor. Repeat three to eleven times. Then, exhale through the nose with ujjayi breathing. Practice seven times.

KRIYAS FOR DHARANA:

NAUMUKI MUDRA

Sit in a meditation position. Keep your eyes closed throughout the exercise. Make sure to have pressure at Mooladhara; use a pillow or blanket if necessary.

Make the khechari mudra and bend your head gently downwards. Mentally repeat "Mooladhara, Mooladhara, Mooladhara." Inhale through the anterior passage to the Bindu. Raise your head as you pass from Vishuddhi to Bindu. Practice shanmuki mudra. Block the ears with the thumbs, the eyes with the index fingers, the nostrils with the middle fingers, the upper lip with the ring fingers, and the lower lip with the little fingers—practice moola bandha and varjoli / sahajoli mudra. Experience the passage along the spine to Bindu. Visualize a trident in copper at the bottom of the Mooladhara. The shaft runs along the spine, and the prongs point upwards from Vishuddhi. The trident rises spontaneously several times, and its middle prong pierces Bindu. When it penetrates Bindu, you mentally say "Bindu bhedan". After a while, release the varjoli / sahajoli mudra and moola bandha and drop your hands on your knees—Exhale from the Bindu with ujjayi breathing along the posterior passage and down to the Mooladhara. Say "Mooladhara, Mooladhara, Mooladhara," mentally. Repeat the exercise. Practice five rounds and finish by exhaling.

SHAKTI CHALINI

Sit in a meditation position. Keep your eyes closed throughout the exercise. Practice khechari mudra. Exhale completely, tilt your head forward, and experience Mooladhara. Repeat mentally, "Mooladhara, Mooladhara, Mooladhara," and then ascend along the front passage to Bindu with ujjayi breathing. Lift your head when you reach Bindu. Hold your breath and practice shanmukhi mudra. Let the consciousness flow continuously down the back passage and up along the front passage while holding your breath. Visualize a narrow green snake moving along the psychic passage. Its head is at Bindu, and it bites its tail. When you follow the snake, you can see how it starts to move along the passage or even make its passages. Look at the snake, no matter what it does. When you need to exhale, release your hands and experience Bindu. Go down the back passage with ujjayi pranayama. Repeat "Mooladhara, Mooladhara, Mooladhara," and ascend along the front passage. Practice five times without interruption.

SHAMBHAVI

Sit in a meditation position. Close your eyes and practice khechari mudra. Visualize a lotus flower with a long green stalk extending downwards. The roots are white or transparent green. The roots spread outwards from the Mooladhara chakra. The lotus flower is at the Sahasrara chakra and is closed like a bud. At the bottom of the bud are some light green leaves. The fallen petals of the flower are pink with delicate red veins. Try to see the lotus. You visualize it in chidakasha and feel it all over your body. Exhale and take consciousness to the root of the Mooladhara chakra. Inhale with ujjayi breathing and let your consciousness rise along the stem upwards along the spine. At the end of inhalation, you reach the bud of the flower. Keep your attention on the Sahasrara and hold your breath. You are inside the lotus flower but can also see it outside. It begins to unfold slowly. When the flower opens, you can see its yellow pollen sprinkled in the middle. The lotus closes and opens almost immediately again. When the lotus has stopped opening and closing, exhale with ujjayi and go down the stem to the Mooladhara. Stay there and experience how the roots spread in different directions. Repeat the exercise eleven times.

AMRIT PAN

Sit in a meditation position. Keep one eye closed and practice khechari mudra. Take consciousness to the Manipura chakra. A warm, sweet liquid is stored there. Exhale completely with ujjayi while taking a quantity of fluid to the Vishuddhi chakra along the spine. Stay at Vishuddhi for a while. The liquid that you brought with you from Manipura is now cooled down. With ujjayi breathing, you exhale up to the Lalana chakra. Inflate the cold fluid up to the Lalana chakra using the breath. Take consciousness to the Manipura chakra again. Repeat the exercise nine times.

CHAKRA BHEDAN

Sit in a meditation position. Keep your eyes closed throughout the exercise. Practice khechari mudra and ujjayi pranayama. Breathe without interruption between inhaling and exhaling. Exhale and take consciousness to the Swadhisthana chakra. Inhale, bring consciousness to the Mooladhara chakra and up along the anterior passage. At Vishuddhi kshetram, breathing will end, and you will start exhaling immediately. Exhale from Vishuddhi kshetram to Bindu and then down the spine from Ajna to Swadhisthana chakra. It is a complete round. Practice fifty-nine rounds. If you become too introverted, finish the exercise and move on to the next kriya.

SUSHUMNA DARSHAN

Sit in a meditation position, close your eyes, and breathe normally. Take consciousness to the Mooladhara chakra. Imagine a pencil with which you draw a square at the Mooladhara chakra. Draw an inverted triangle inside the square. Then, make a circle that touches each corner of the square. Make four petals on each side of the square. Take consciousness to Swadhisthana. Draw a circle there as big as the previous one. Draw six petals around the circle and a crescent moon inside it. Take consciousness to Manipura. Draw a circle and draw an inverted triangle inside it. In the middle of it, you draw a fireball.

Make ten petals around the circle. Take consciousness to the Anahata. Draw two triangles that lie on each other, one with the tip up and the other with the tip down. Draw a circle around these with twelve petals. Then, take consciousness to Vishuddhi. Draw a circle with a smaller circle inside, like a drop of nectar. Make sixteen petals around the circle. Take consciousness to the eye. Draw a circle with the sign Om inside. Draw two large petals around the circle, one on the right and one on the left. For Bindu, draw a crescent moon with a small circle above it. At Sahasrara, make a circle with a triangle with the tip facing up. There are a thousand petals around the circle. Try to see all the chakras in their respective places. It can be challenging to see everything at once, so start by visiting two at a time and adding a new one for each day.

PRANA AHUTI

Sit in a meditation position. Close your eyes and breathe normally. Experience a light pressure on the top of the head, the pressure of a divine hand. The hand provides the body and mind with prana flowing down from the Sahasrara along the spine. You may experience this as cold, heat, electricity, or a stream of liquid or wind. When the prana has reached the Mooladhara chakra, you go directly to the next kriya.

UTTHAN

Sit in a meditation position. Close your eyes and breathe normally. Take consciousness to the Mooladhara chakra. Try to visualize it as detailed as you can. See a black Shiva lingam. The bottom of the lingam is cut away, and a small red snake moves around it. The snake tries to entangle itself so it can rise along the sushumna. While it struggles to eliminate it, it makes an angry hissing sound. The tail is attached to the Shiva lingam, but the body and head rise along the spine and then come down again. You may experience this as the body contracts, followed by happiness and bliss. When this occurs, move on to the next kriya.

SWAROOPA DARSHAN

Sit in a meditation position and keep your eyes closed. Become aware of your physical body. Your body is entirely still. You are as solid as a mountain. Become aware of your natural breathing while ensuring your body is completely still. Your body solidifies and becomes immobile. After a while, you are absorbed by the natural breath while your body thickens. When your body is so still that you cannot move it even though you want to, you move on to the next kriya.

LINGA SANCHALANA

Sit completely still with your eyes closed. Your breathing has automatically switched to ujjayi breathing, and you are practicing khechari mudra. Be fully aware of your breathing.

With each inhalation, the body expands, and with each exhalation, it contracts. Your physical body is still entirely still; your astral body moves. After a while, you only experience the astral body. You may reach a stage where the astral body, during contraction, becomes a tiny point of light. When this happens, you go straight to the next kriya.

KRIYA FOR DHYANA:

DHYANA

You have experienced your astral body as a tiny point of light. Please look closer at the bright spot and how it resembles a golden egg. When you look at the egg, it begins to expand. It gets the same shape as your astral and physical body as it gets bigger. This form is neither material nor subtle; it is the form of pure light.

This kriya for dhyana can be used as a conclusion in all yoga and all meditations, not only in Kriya yoga.

MAITHUNA

Maithuna, the tantric intercourse within the vamachara tradition, is perhaps the ritual most people associate with tantra. It is known as the most effective method for awakening our dormant, inner cosmic power – Kundalini Shakti. We awaken the Kundalini Shakti in the root chakra – Mooladhara chakra, and guide the energy up through the sushumna nadi along the spine, activating all our chakras. When it reaches the Sahasrara chakra, the crown chakra at the top of our head, we connect to the power of the cosmos and the collective consciousness. Our spine and chakras turn into an antenna that transmits but also receives. The longer we wait to release the orgasm, the stronger the signal becomes and the more power we are filled with. By practicing Maithuna regularly, we gradually become more enlightened.

Historically, the tantrikas of the vamachara tradition used the energy generated from sexual group rituals to obtain siddhis (paranormal / magical powers) and enlightenment. Every woman who participated became a goddess and every man a god. So it was not necessary, exactly, which counterpart one had in the sexual group activity. It was the spiritual experience that mattered and was at the center.

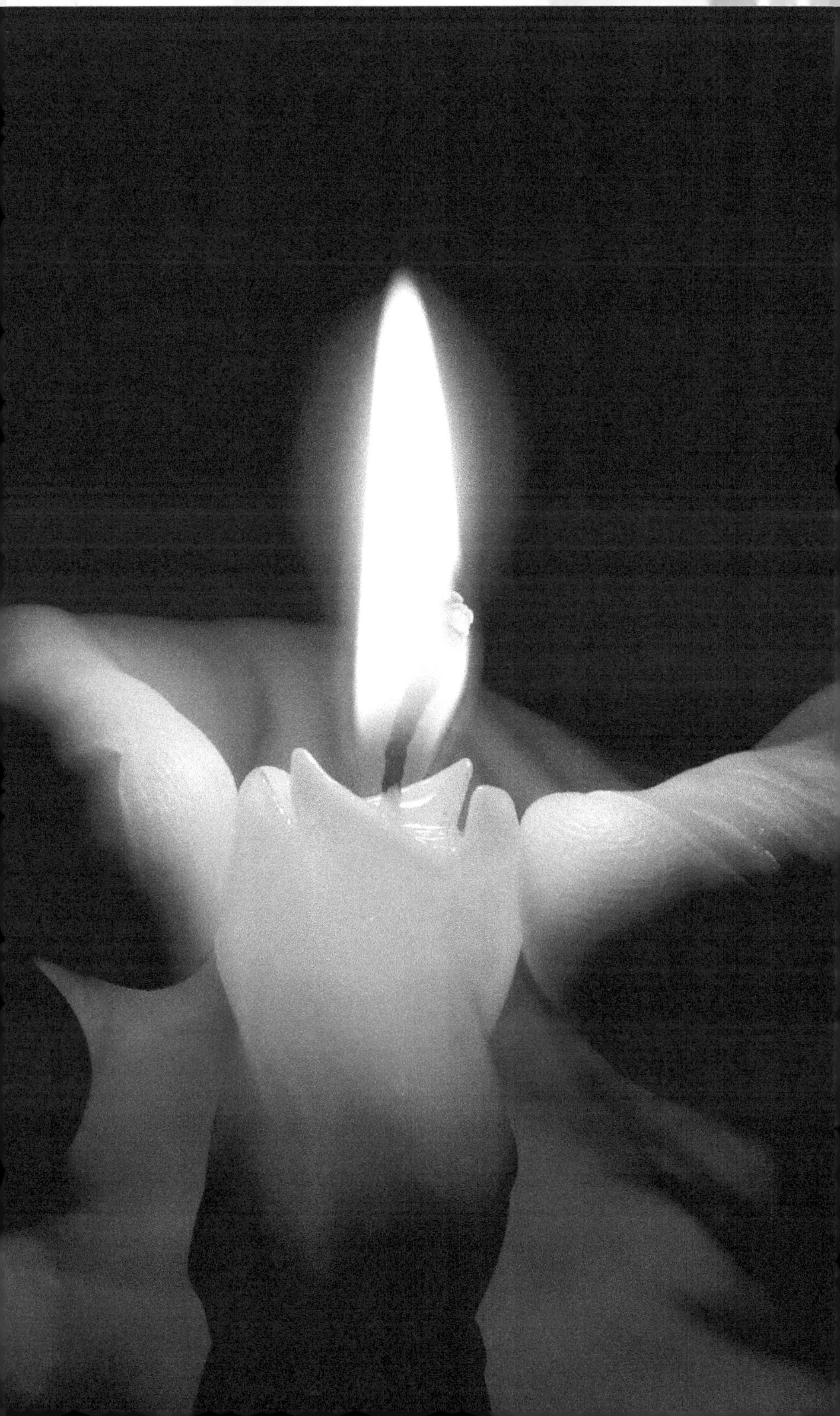

PREPARATION

Everything preceding the act is apt to raise awareness and remove tensions.

1. The room where the ritual occurs is clean; incense should be burned there. The nose and the olfactory organs are connected by nerves and acceptable psychic currents to the Mooladhara chakra, where the Kundalini is twisted. Your attention and sensitivity increase when the sense of smell is affected correctly.

2. Prepare food and flowers to be used during the ritual. The meal consists of four parts, and the room is decorated with flowers.

Pancha makara, tattwa chakra or pancha tattwa is also the name of the five "m" used in the ritual.

Wine – madya.

Wine symbolizes the intoxicating experience of the richness of consciousness achieved through yoga. If you prefer not to use alcohol, you can replace it with non-alcoholic wine or coconut milk. The element fire. Tattwa agni.

Meat – mamsa.

Flesh symbolizes "Everything I am, everything I do and experience – what I stand for, everything is part of my being." If you do not eat meat, replace it with garlic, ginger, sesame seeds, tofu, or other soy products. The element earth. Tattwa prithvi.

Fish – matsya.

Fish symbolizes a state where "I experience everything, the whole universe, pleasure, and pain, as myself. I am all this. I contain all opposites". If you do not eat fish, replace it with aubergines and radishes. The element water. Tattwa apas.

Roasted barley products – mudra.

Rice, wheat, etc. They symbolize that "I stop identifying with fears and inhibitions." The element air. Tattwa vayu.

Flowers (represents intercourse) – maithuna.

Flowers symbolize intercourse, representing the original power, the feminine that rises to the highest chakra and unites with the masculine. The element space. Tattwa akasha.

3. Shower together. It is relaxing, invigorating, and prepares you both to meet your "divine partner." Shakti (the woman who symbolizes all women) is lubricated with fragrant oils and perfumes. Different oils can be rubbed into other body parts, such as musk oil around the Venus mountain.

Then, you especially massage your partner's spine. Start at the lower part of the spine, press your thumbs alternately with small movements back and forth, and work your way up along the spine. The area where the sushumna, ida, and pingala nadi flow is then released from tension and activated.

TO OPEN UP

The room has been decorated with flowers, the food has been served, and the wine has been poured; incense glows, candles are burning, or even better, an oil lamp that emits a red glow.

The next step in this holy experience is to inaugurate and cleanse the room and the house by sprinkling water and saying a mantra. A mantra with long lines of verse is usually used.

This part of the ritual is extensive and precisely laid out to keep the mind occupied. The mind comes in an elevated and secure state. Here, you can use the mantra – Am Hrim Krom Hamsah So-Ham, repeated aloud eleven times. To the house or surroundings, to the room, to those present, to the food, to the wine, to the four directions, up and down. The different bija mantras are often translated as other manifestations of energy and consciousness. In this context, however, the mantra represents "conscious attention."

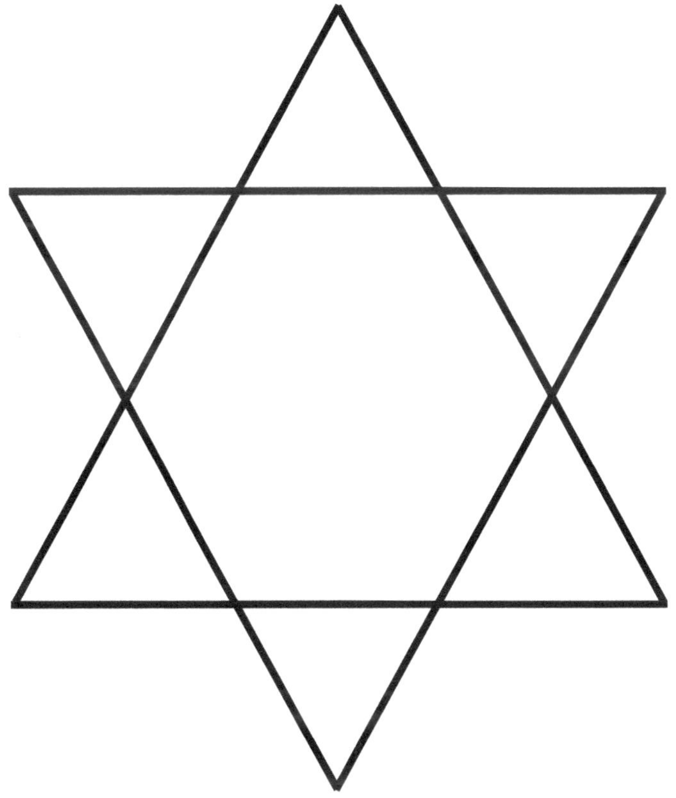

The two triangles symbolize the female and male parts of the universe. Shiva and Shakti. Purusha and Prakriti. Consciousness and energy.

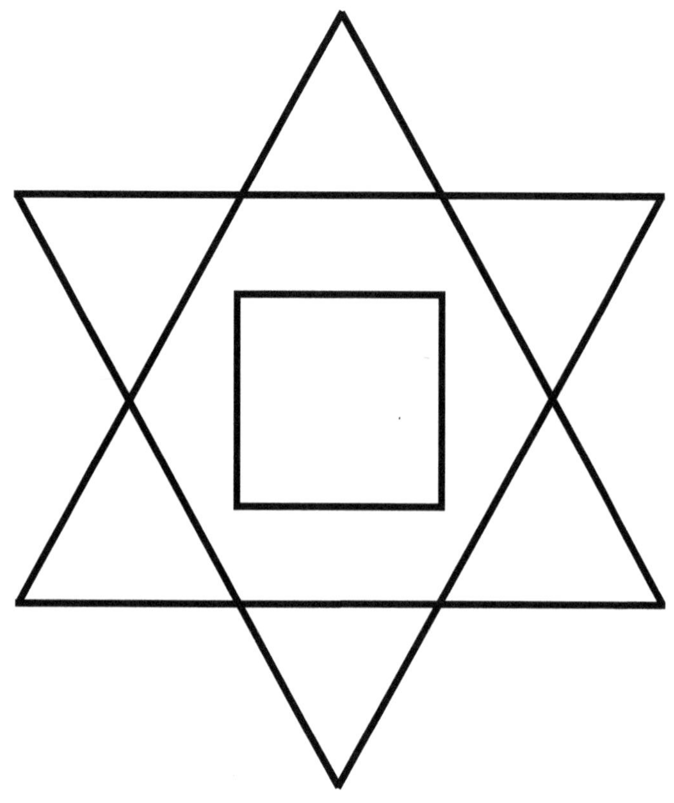

The square symbolizes the foundation from which the power is aroused and rises, the Mooladhara chakra.

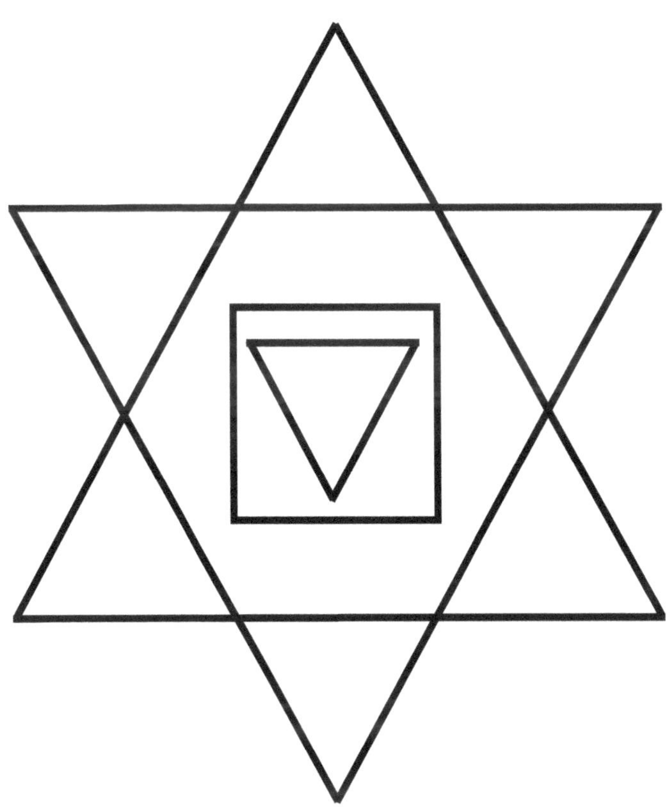

The force, Kundalini, is symbolized by the last triangle.

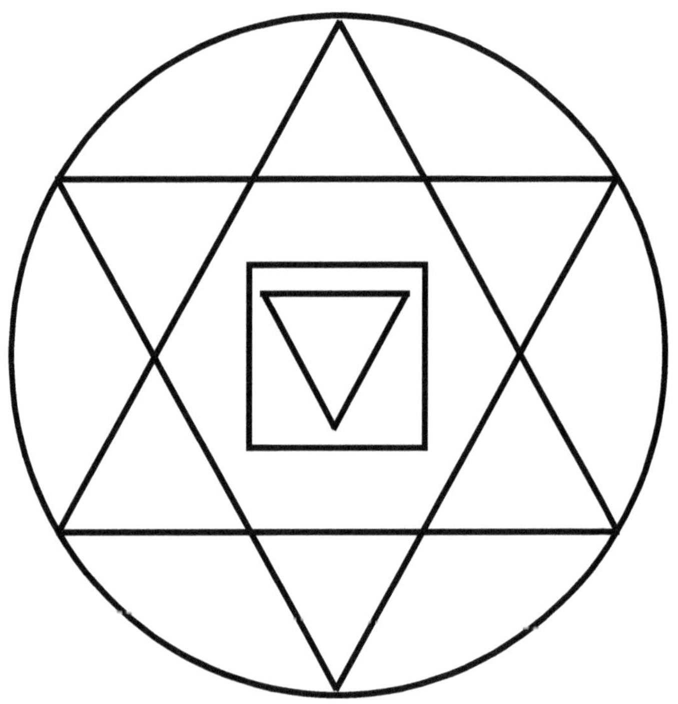

The circle symbolizes eternity.

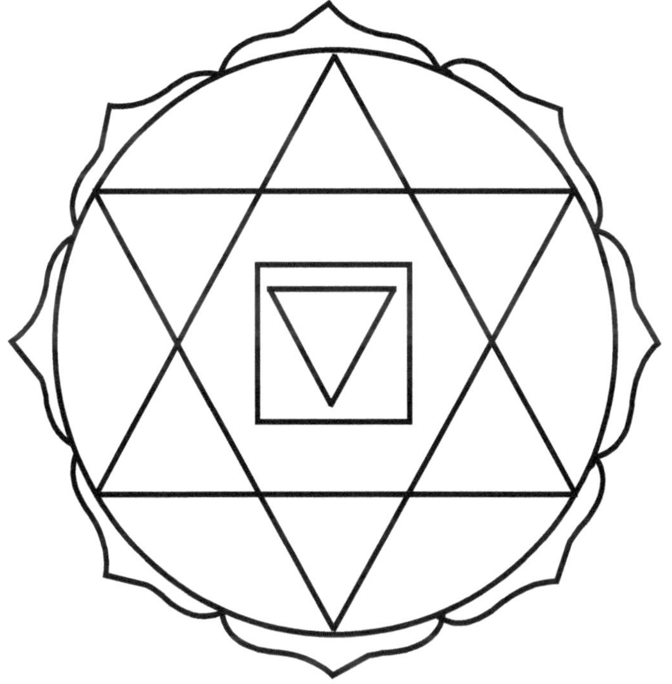

The petals symbolize infinity.

Have a small bowl of water in front of you, dip your fingers in it, sprinkle the water as above, and say the mantra Swaha (I burn it, I donate it) each time. Also, dip some flowers in the water and throw them on the food – Swaha, on the wine – Swaha, on those present – Swaha ...

This act should last so long and thorough that you become wholly preoccupied with it and can indulge in it seriously and without reservation.

With his finger dipped in red powder mixed with a bit of soapy water and oil, Shakti puts a red dot in the center of the eyebrows of those present. She also gets a point. It symbolizes the ability for concentration and empathy achieved through the Ajna chakra in the middle of the head. If Ajna's chakra is aroused, you will participate in this act without tension, without being hampered by shame or frivolity.

YOGA AND MEDITATION

Do pranayamas and bandhas and yoga nidra. Then, use the So-Ham (or your mantra) with ujjayi pranayama. Meditate with So-Ham – So as you inhale, and Ham as you exhale. So-Ham means, "I am that – I am part of the divine, I am God." Meditate on your body. Experience your natural breathing until you reach a deep and calm state, then repeat the mental mantra Am Hrim Krom Hamsah So-Ham. Experience your body as light – imagine that the body is made of pure light and that this light destroys every fear in you, every inhibition, and all hatred. Experience that you are prepared for the cosmic act. You experience the union between the power – the feminine in you, and the consciousness – the masculine. Experience a strengthening and cleansing light flow that fills your body and breathing.

RITUALS

A guru is appointed to lead the ritual if several people are present. He dips his middle finger in the water and draws a downward-pointing triangle on the floor where you sit, and then over this, he draws an upward-pointing triangle. In the middle of both triangles – in the middle of the hexagonal star, draw a smaller square and, in the square, another downward-pointing triangle. A circle that touches all the corners is drawn around both triangles; then, eight petals are drawn around the outside of the circle.

The two triangles symbolize the female and male parts of the universe. Shiva and Shakti. Purusha and Prakriti. Consciousness and energy. The square symbolizes the foundation from which the power is aroused and rises, the Mooladhara chakra. The force, Kundalini, is represented by the last triangle. The circle symbolizes eternity. The petals symbolize infinity.

Finally, before the action itself, an essential part of the ritual comes: the wine is inaugurated by Shakti with flowers, water, and the mantra Swaha. She opens the wine to everyone present. The wine has a liberating effect on the mind, but do not drink too much. Consciousness must pass clearly.

The man sits in a meditation position. The woman sits on his left thigh. They give each other wine and food, feeding each other. If this position is too difficult, you can sit beside each other with the woman seated to the man's left.

Just as scents affect Mooladhara chakra, Swadhisthana chakra is affected by food and drink. All this increases the desire and sensitivity.

THE ACT

Sit opposite your partner – look each other in the eyes. You are entirely naked – two people, a man and a woman, and experience each other's sex and desire. You appreciate each other; two divine beings participate in a universal action.

Meditate on each other, and experience each other with desire and joy. If you smile from embarrassment or tense muscles in your face or body, return to the relaxed naturalness every time. Get back to the game and the seriousness of what you do repeatedly. If limiting thoughts arise – whatever happens, accept it and then return to the experience of each other.

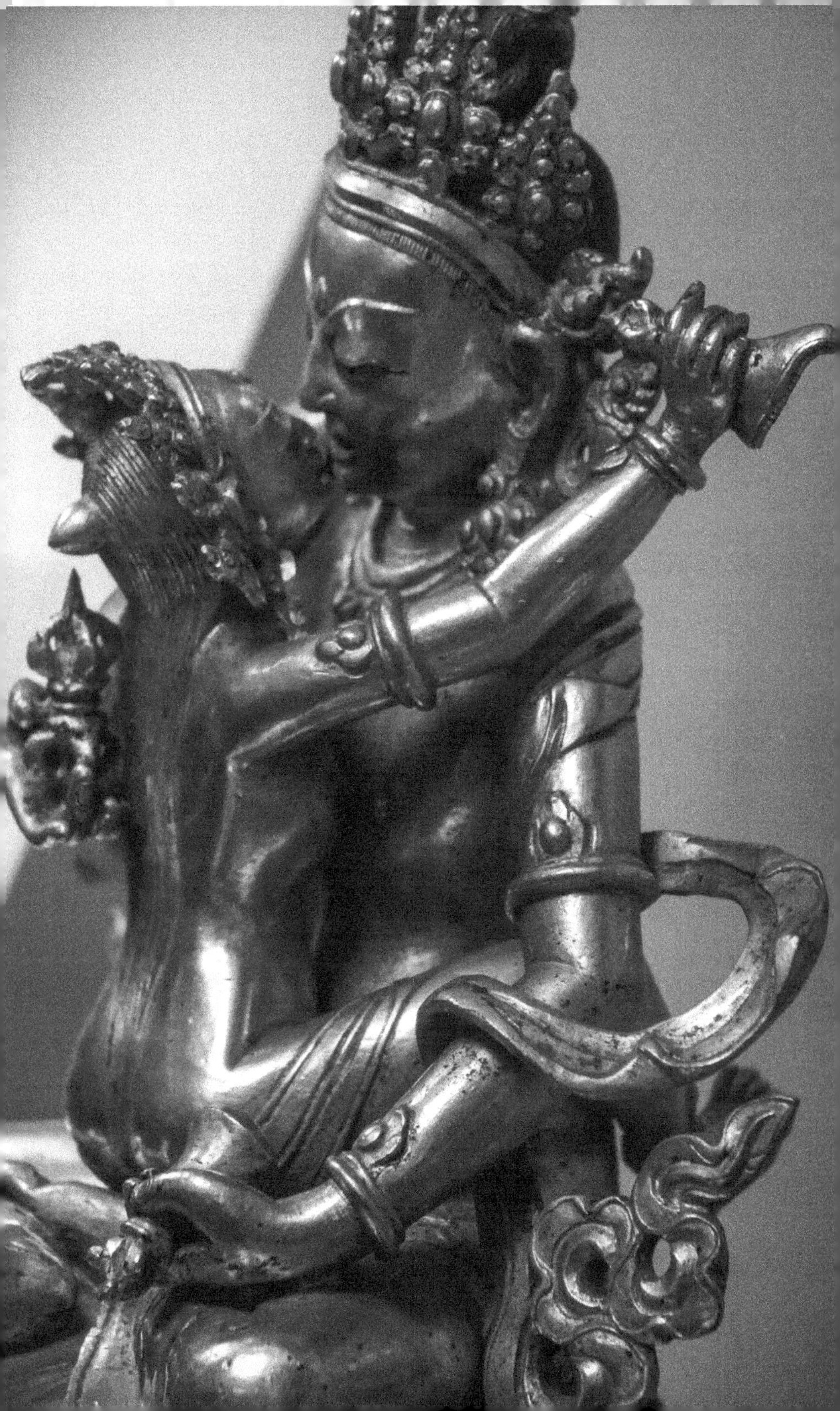

Continue to experience your divine partner for a long time. You do not have to demand, explain, or excuse anything. You should not achieve anything – be, experience, enjoy!

The intercourse itself can be performed either in the following way or in one of the sixty-four tantric positions. In the tantric positions, you take a sexual yoga position. It is not done mechanically or by you getting up and sitting down again; it is done without losing touch with each other, even for a second. Remain immobile in every position ...

POSITIONS

1. The man sits in a meditation position, and the woman sits down on the man and wraps her legs around the man's waist and hips so that her feet are crossed behind his seat.

2. Same as 1 – but instead of the woman crossing her legs behind him, she lifts them while the man holds his arms under her knees and embraces her around the waist and lower back.

3. The man is lying on his back, and the woman is squatting on him.

4. The woman starts by sitting as in 3, then lies backward between the man's legs and stretches her legs along his body.

5. Standing. The man stands on the floor and holds the woman while she hangs on him with her legs and arms wrapped around him.

6. The woman lies stretched out on the man or vice versa. There are several variations; the back must be straight or in the yoga position. Remain immobile in the position while you experience each other mentally and physically. Together, you go into an uninterrupted sexual meditation. You are immobile. The experience of mental and physical union can come at any time, and when it comes, stay in it as long as it is at its peak, then end it.

The shortest time in a position is more than half an hour to reach any fundamental transformation.

However, you do not have to worry about the body or the performance; let the Shakti in your partner lead you and your inspiration. Give and receive. Do not strive for a normal orgasm, but let the experience of each other transform you. The sixty-four positions symbolize freedom from expectations so you can do things differently each time. You decide for yourself.

Get used to the ritual; do it many times. Gradually, you will master it and get the full benefit of it. It will have a more profound effect when it can be done effortlessly.

In addition to the ritual performed by a couple, there are rituals shared by several couples sitting together in a circle. The introductory part of the ritual is performed by all couples together. The woman chosen to be Shakti for all present in the circle symbolizes power and is honored to be one. She pours the wine, leads the serving of the food, and thus begins the ritual. A guru performs the mantra ritual and guides the meditation and the process. During intercourse itself, in the different positions, each pair sits separately in a large circle called the chakra. The feast or ritual that raises consciousness is called puja – chakra puja.

Meditating with others creates a strong force field and supports everyone who participates. There are different puja: In the Bharai chakra, you have a partner appointed in advance. In yogini puja, you choose freely and independently of the individual.

A chakra puja can be done in different ways. Having intercourse as a ritual is so crucial that it can have a liberating effect on our lives. It becomes a beautiful and central act in human society.

SEX MAGIC

Sexual power and orgasm create life and are the most vital energy in the cosmos. Therefore, it is used in yoga, tantra, and magic to give the practitioner the ultimate power. It is logical and easy to understand.

After initiating sexual magic, you become a magician. The initiation takes place from man to woman and from woman to man. The guru – regardless of gender, passes on his magical powers to the adept via Shaktipat. The adept is initiated with the guru's orgasm.

Even if you do not possess the magical power of a magician, you can use your sexual magic rituals to get what you want, such as supernatural desire.

MAGICAL WISH

1. Write down / draw your wish on paper or use a picture of what you wish. Put it next to you and say the wish out loud to yourself.

2. Start masturbating and experience an inner image of desire in the Mooladhara chakra—experience how the image is in the chakra and turns dark red. Experience four petals that enclose the image.

3. Experience how you draw the image of the Swadhisthana chakra, how it turns orange, and how six petals enclose it.

4. Experience how you draw the image of the Manipura chakra, how it turns yellow, and how ten petals enclose it.

5. Experience how you draw the image to the Anahata chakra, how the picture turns blue, and how twelve petals enclose it.

6. Experience how you draw the image to the Vishuddhi chakra, how it becomes violet in color, and how sixteen petals enclose it.

7. Experience how you draw the image to the Ajna chakra, how the image turns white, and how the shape of a pyramid encloses it.

8. Experience how you draw the image to the Sahasrara chakra, how it turns purple-red, and how an infinite number of petals enclose it.

9. When the orgasm comes, you shoot the image out of the Sahasrara chakra, and you mentally experience how the desire leaves the scalp and goes away into the cosmos.

If you change after making your magical wish, you will burn up the image of the want so that it ceases to work.

Did you like the book? Feel free to follow me on my social media, share and like, tell your friends about the books, and feel free to write an honest review; one or two lines don't matter. All support is precious. Thanks!

On my Facebook page and Instagram, I post exciting news and tips on temporary offers and benefits you can take advantage of. I often also post my yoga routine and other things related to nutrition and health that may be interesting to take part in. So feel free to join them so you don't miss anything interesting:

 *facebook.com/bhagwanoneofakindbooks*

 *instagram.com/bhagwanoneofakindbooks/*

MY BOOKS AND BOOK SERIES

I have two book series that have different audiences. Great Yoga Books – is a series with the most comprehensive fact books on yoga for those who want to explore the subject in depth. Here, you will also find classic yoga books that are rarely translated, such as Patanjali's Yoga Sutras and Hatha Yoga Pradipika. My second series, Yoga Beyond the Poses: The Ultimate Beginner's Guide to Yoga, covers one yoga topic at a time and is extra easy to read with larger text. For those who find it challenging to read extensive books and want a good and broad overview of the subject quickly. Both series are also available as audiobooks.

★★★★★

TEACHING YOGA
&
MEDITATION
BEYOND
THE POSES

BESTSELLING AUTHOR

Shreyananda Natha

Teaching Yoga and Meditation Beyond the Poses – A unique and practical workbook!

Teaching Yoga and Meditation Beyond the Poses – A unique and practical workbook for aspiring yoga teachers who want to teach yoga and meditation beyond the poses.

Teaching Yoga and Meditation Beyond the Poses is a unique and essential resource for new and experienced teachers and a guide for all yoga students interested in refining their skills and knowledge. Teaching Yoga and Meditation is also ideal as a core textbook in yoga teacher training programs.

The book covers fundamental yoga philosophy and history topics, including a historical presentation of classical yoga literature: Yoga Sutras of Patanjali, Bhagavad Gita, etc. Each of the seven major styles of yoga is described, from Hatha yoga, Raja yoga, Tantra yoga, Bhakti yoga, and Kundalini yoga, to knowledge about the chakras, Ayurveda and magic mantras and yantras. The book provides extensive support and tools for teaching integrated and classical yoga (asanas), breathing techniques (pranayama), deep relaxation (Yoga Nidra), and meditation (Ajapa Japa). The book is divided into eight modules with associated knowledge tests and complete yoga and meditation classes.

https://rb.gy/9s6edj

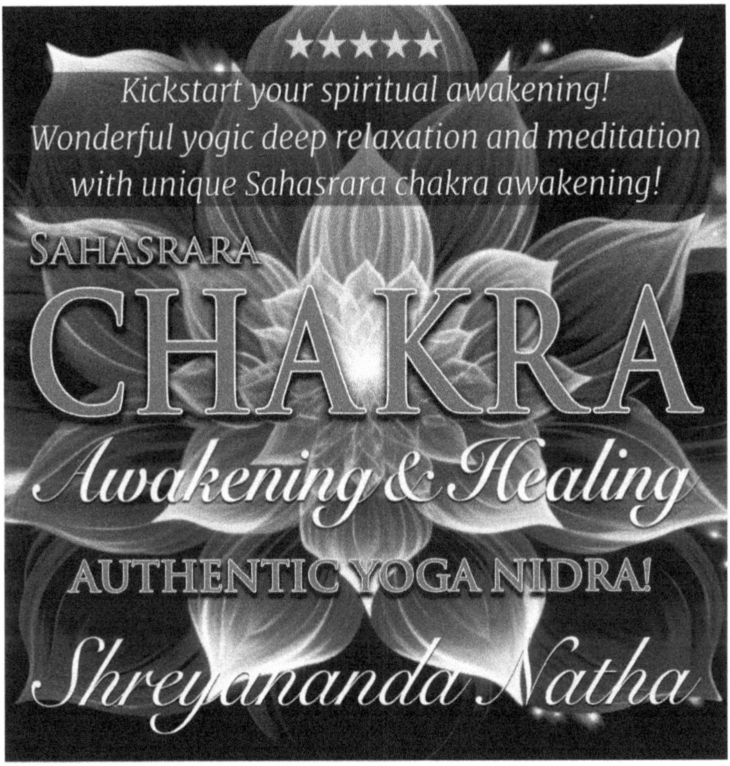

Download the **AUDIOBOOK** here!

SCAN QR-CODE or go to:

https://bit.ly/47MSQ81